*T*

# RUNNING in CHURCH

**CAN'T COUNT FOR CARDIO!**

# RUNNING in CHURCH

## CAN'T COUNT FOR CARDIO!

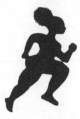

**12** *Practical Prayers* **TO IGNITE** *Your Weight Loss Journey*

## QUEING JONES

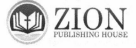
ZION
PUBLISHING HOUSE

*To all the women who promise to love themselves in their before, during, and after stages.*

*You are enough.*

# *FOREWORD*

Dr. Anitra Shelton-Quinn

In life, coming in contact with people who are movers and shakers, that impact the community to bring about positive change is an invaluable commodity. Whenever I have the opportunity to sit down and talk with author, Queing Jones, the passion and power radiating from her experiential journey is life-giving. From encouraging the masses by sharing testimonial tidbits of her amazing journey of health and wellness, to pouring out words of wisdom to foster positive change, Queing's transparency and "realness" lends to the world, a voice of truth and triumph. Giving rise to this biblically sound self-help guide, Jones masterfully guides readers through a heart-to-heart, conversational literary journey. Drawing from the hills and valleys of her considerable weight-loss, time in the trenches of health and wellness, and her deep-rooted passion to reach people with a God-inspired mission, Queing's message equips others to live healthy and well. Wrapped in biblical truths with practical strategies, Queing gives readers the sure-fire tools for a successful weight-loss journey.

As a psychologist of twenty years, with extensive training and experience in behavior change, I am all too familiar with the rollercoaster of motivation and meaningful change, often rooted in the psychological trauma and spiritual conflict, that often impedes success on the road to a healthy lifestyle. Specifically, according to the American Psychological Association (APA), a major aspect of weight control involves understanding & managing thoughts and behaviors that can interfere with weight-loss. A variety of issues that influence weight gain, such as stress, anxiety, depression, low-self-esteem, illness, injuries, and past abuse or trauma are examples of how issues can influence emotional eating and associated weight gain. At the end of the day, as a psychologist, I subscribe the ideology that sustained weight-loss isn't about strict dieting, but a more holistic approach to both body and mind.

A nationally recognized expert in the field of psychology—having presented amongst some of the greatest intellectual minds across the nation, including the National Association of School Psychologists (NASP), the Association of Behavior Analysis (ABA) International Convention, National Alliance of Mental Illness (NAMI), and the Gerontological Society of America (GSA) National Convention, and a mouthpiece for the most high God, as author of "Becoming Incredibly Irresistible" (Christian Self-Help Bestseller), I count it an honor and a privilege to compose the foreword for this literary, self-help masterpiece. Unlike other quick-fix diet plans, "Running in Church Can't Count as Cardio," empowers readers through "real-life" lessons, to tap into God's power through His Word and prayer to lose the weight, once and for all, and keep it off. The faith and fortitude that Queing conveys through her message and her life, epitomizes the transformative power found in God's Word and His grace. Finally, given the grave public health threat that obesity poses, with links to chronic diseases, including high blood pressure, cardiovascular disease, and cancer, it is my prayer that this book extends a lifeline to those struggling to live a healthy, abundant life, for the glory of God.

# MY TRANSFORMATION STORY

My weight-loss journey has been off and on since I was a freshman in college, thinking I was "fat," when I was actually fine. And, like some of you, I would have success losing ten, twenty, or thirty or so pounds, but I'd gain it all back again. Then, I'd do nothing for another year or decade. It wasn't until the summer of 2014, when I put a stake in the ground and committed myself to going all the way through the process this time.

I've been asked where my motivation came from. Looking back, I can see that it was birthed out of a very broken place. I felt so hopeless in so many areas of my life. Through Godly counsel from sister friends (and also listening to inspirational teachings), I decided that I would be more compassionate with myself and treat *me* as if I were my own best friend. I would be good to myself in every way. That included the way I talked to myself about myself and the way that I cared for my body.

I started with just walking. This was good for my body and my soul because I would use that time to pray and plan. After a couple of months of walking, I noticed some ladies who were working out together in the park. I stopped to talk to them and learned they had been training together for a while. I got the meet-up information from their trainer and promised to follow-up about joining them. About a month or so later, I actually did follow up, and I began working out with them three times a week. I started to really enjoy group training. Before this time, I did not understand the benefits of strength training, which was a component of these workouts. Now, my body was beginning to transform beyond weight loss, as I was gaining endurance AND muscle! I worked out with that group throughout the fall, and by the beginning of winter, I was down twenty pounds.

At the start of 2015, I discovered a fitness boutique that specialized in weight training for women, *Dre's Diesel Dome (D3)*, in Chicago. I came to D3 looking to take my body beyond where I could transform it on my own. I was struggling to break the two-hundred-pound mark. Well, after only a month at D3, I lost thirteen pounds and was well under two hundred pounds for the first time in over a decade! What I discovered was that the training, nutritional education, and sisterhood at D3 is what I had been missing. These tools offered by D3 helped to radically transform my understanding of fitness and also inspired my personal mission to encourage other women to begin or renew their own fitness journeys.

Before I was living a fit life, my diet was dominated by fast food, junk food, processed foods (stuff out of a bag, box, or can), and occasionally even so-called healthy foods, which were actually far from healthy. The alleged "healthy foods" were high in sodium and/or sugars and very low in quality protein. When I started to eat less of the mess, I would have some success. However, I would sabotage those good efforts by overeating on the weekends, then I would attempt to start all over again every Monday.

Through following weight blogs and success stories, I learned about clean eating. I even did my own *Google* research on it. I realized eating clean needed to be my next step if I wanted to get stronger inside and out. I chose

19

more whole foods that I prepared at home—whole grains, fruits, vegetables, beans, chicken breast, etc. Foods that have not been processed to death! I chose to keep foods as close to their natural form as possible, basically without all the additives and preservatives. That's when I started seeing changes which became lasting. I lost more weight in my first three months of clean eating and working out than I had in the entire time with poor eating and working out! It's true. You can't outrun a bad diet.

My advice for anyone who wants to lose weight is to start with cultivating a greater love for yourself. When you love someone, you want to give them your absolute best. The same goes for our own selves. When we love ourselves tremendously, we will be willing to be patient and compassionate with ourselves throughout the process. I would also encourage you to have a personal declaration, mantra, or scripture for daily motivation.

My daily motivation is 1 Corinthians 9:27 (MSG), "I don't know about you, but I'm running hard for the finish line. I'm giving it everything I've got. No sloppy living for me! I'm staying alert and in top condition. I'm not going to get caught napping, telling everyone else all about it and then missing out myself."

I was heavy for over twenty years —overweight in my 20's, obese in my 30's, now I'm getting fit in my 40's! Friend, if you're reading this, know you, too have what it takes to do this once and for all! And, you will! Remember this—be merciful and compassionate toward yourself along the way. We will get there together!

**Our Churches Are Filled with Big Believers! Literally.**

**So, a lot (a whole lot) of people of faith are overweight or obese**. People of faith are more likely to be overweight than people who identify as non-religious. This is according to some longitudinal studies (studies done repeatedly over time) by both Northwestern University and Purdue

University[1]. The findings also show folks who attend church more frequently are actually twice as likely to become obese than those who are less involved in church-related activities. That's crazy, right! Interesting but not surprising. And, as we look around our congregations, church leaders and those working in ministry are struggling as well. A study by *Pulpit and Pew*, which provides research on pastoral leadership, revealed that 76% of clergy were overweight or obese compared with 61% of the general church-goer population. Enough with the statistics.

---

[1] *Religious Young Adults Become Obese by Middle Age.* Northwestern University, Feinberg School of Medicine. 2011. Retrieved on February 27, 2019 from: https://www.northwestern.edu/newscenter/stories/2011/03/religious-young-adults-obese.html.

You get the point. It's an important point for us to acknowledge.

My own personal theory of why this is so is that the culture of some churches centers around food as THE main way to fellowship. And, that is a wonderful way to fellowship, so that's not what I'm saying. We see in the scriptures that believers would often "break bread" together after being taught or as part of a celebration. However, whereas they may have had lean meats, vegetables, and fruit. We, on the other hand, might be having fried chicken, ribs, mac and cheese, corn bread, banana pudding, pound cake, and fruit punch. And, all that might even go down right there in the church. We do see more progressive churches being very innovative with how they fellowship and celebrate, so I believe we are turning those unhealthy traditions around. Slowly but surely.

Another reason for those statistics could be connected to how there are some of us who have believed that focusing on our bodies is vain or even selfish. You probably have heard, "God looks on the heart" (1 Samuel 16:7) used almost as an excuse for complacency. And, yes, He does see our hearts. Yet, the Word also says that physical training has some benefits, too (1 Timothy 4:8). It's good for us. It is not more important than spiritual training, but it is important. If we struggle with considering that we can successfully train our bodies to eat cleaner and to have endurance with exercise (1 Corinthians 9:27), or if we are challenged with acknowledging our own beauty (Psalm 139:14) when we are in fact God's masterpiece (Ephesians 2:10), then we can easily slip into settling for a physical state that we criticize more than we celebrate. And, that is exactly what I did for most of my teen years and adult life. Even though, I could have believed for better.

As believers, we can be so intentional with applying our faith in many different areas of our lives. This is a good thing! Whether it's for a new job, a new apartment or house, an increase in income, clarity in a relationship, peace for our communities, good weather, justice, approval, or a parking space...you name it! We pray for it, get agreement on it, march around it, declare it, high-five our neighbor, sow a seed for it, or whatever else we feel led to do as an act of faith. And, all that matters. So, why are we slack on activating these high levels of faith in the area of nutrition and fitness? I had to ask this of myself.

See, I thought I *was* applying my faith in my weight loss efforts during my on-again off-again diet attempts. But, really what I was doing was just praying to God to help me lose weight but not taking smart, consistent actions that were in line with my goals. I was only responding emotionally to my physical condition. Then, I'd give up and try again. And, again and again; all the while gaining back whatever I lost and then some. I'm hoping, as believers, we can confront and challenge how we apply our faith to our physical health and prioritize like we do with other areas of our lives.

*Beloved, I pray that in every way you may succeed and prosper and be in good health [physically], just as [I know] your soul prospers [spiritually].*
*III John 1:2 (AMP)*

I believe weight loss is indeed a spiritual endeavor. Losing one hundred and two pounds was one of the greatest adventures of my life and certainly one of the most intense. My journey continues, as I am now navigating my way through maintenance, which for me has been significantly more challenging than the initial weight loss. But, one thing remains constant-prayer. Praying regarding weight loss, as part of your overall desire to prosper in health, is a divine idea. It is not vain or prideful to want to be in optimal health and to feel good about the way you look along the way.

Over the next twelve days, I will share with you some scriptures and prayer confessions to help you reset your thinking and "fan the fires" of your faith as it relates to your weight loss journey. Whether you are just starting out, starting over, almost at your goal, somewhere in the middle, or mastering maintenance, you can benefit from these short but power-packed spiritual exercises. If you're on social media, use the hashtag #runninginchurch to connect and share your experience with the community of believers on this journey with you.

## How to Get the Most Out of This Experience

- Take your time with the readings and prayers. Move on when you feel you've got that day's lesson locked into your spirit. It's okay to spend multiple days or a week or more on just one of the days. If you'd like, you can read all the way through, and then start over with a focus on meditating on the lessons more thoroughly.

- Consider writing out the prayers and placing them in a binder to go back to for reflection. Please also consider writing your own prayer confessions and posting them up at home in your most frequented spots.

- Consider this a resource for whenever you need a boost. This is a living document. When you read it again, you will discover something new.

- Most importantly, come into this with the mindset that this is not a formula and neither is it magic. Instead, this is you literally exercising your faith.

# DAY ONE
## TRANSFORMATION IS AN INSIDE JOB!

It's Day One! Y'all, if I had tallied all the times I lost weight and gained every ounce of it back, it would be a double-digit number for sure. See, I thought by following a formula—"Eat this not that," "Workout like this not that"—I'd lose the weight for good, and I would be much happier. Bless my heart. I was starting with the physical, when I should have been starting with the spiritual. Because, just eating the "right" foods and working out never seemed to be enough. If you're reading this book, you can probably relate.

What I overlooked through many failed attempts, is that my issues with my weight were much deeper than understanding the glycemic index or HIIT (high intensity interval training). What took me a long time to come to terms with is that **weight loss is, above all else, a spiritual endeavor.** A wisdom principle I have learned is transformation should follow an impact pattern of: SPIRIT, SOUL, MIND, and BODY. But, out of our eagerness for change, we approach it starting with a focus on just the physical (BODY). We become frustrated and eventually quit. The next time we go after weight loss, we try again with a new level of understanding, and we add MIND to it. This means we learn more about nutrition and fitness and begin to apply that knowledge more intentionally.

We go further this time, but when life sucker-punches us, we get distracted and thrown off course. When we do overcome, we often find ourselves more overweight. But, we're not quitters! So, we try again, and this time we have progressed from that set back, so we have SOUL, MIND, and BODY operating. We are affirming ourselves, loving ourselves, recognizing and dismantling negative self-talk, and are more motivated than ever before. And, this takes us even further, perhaps to finally reaching our ultimate weight-loss goal and maintaining it for quite some time.

At this level, it can be difficult to distinguish that we need something more. However, we may come to discover a whole other set of anxieties. For example, I remember feeling like a stranger in my new body. Other times, I felt in bondage or resentful about having to be so mindful of my eating and workouts. I didn't feel free. I was enjoying the results but not the process. I didn't know I would wake up one day and not want to do any of it anymore nor would I have the grace to do it. So, much of what I was doing was in my own strength and will power.

I am so grateful the Lord graced me with the desire to try yet again, but this time starting with SPIRIT. I've come to delightfully discover that feeding my spirit empowers my SOUL (emotions, character, perception), re-freshes and inspires my MIND (thinking, intellect, choices), and even impacts my physical BODY. It's an inside-out transformation. That's what is available to us—the opportunity to be spirit-led in our weight loss journey. This matters so much because until we release our emotional and mental weight, the physical weight will continue to slither back on over time, no matter how many times we think we've let it go for good. Even if we maintain our weight loss for life, it will be burdensome to have a dream body with an anxious soul and easily agitated mind.

I've learned the hard way, the longer way, that formulas (weight loss programs, diets and meal plans, pills and powders, gyms, trainers and boot-camps, etc.) won't solve the problem we're experiencing with being consistent with self-control. On Day One, let's ask the Lord to reset our thinking to approach weight loss starting at the SPIRIT level.

### Romans 12:2 (MSG)

*So, here's what I want you to do, God helping you: Take your everyday, ordinary life—your sleeping, eating, going-to-work, and walking-around life—and place it before God as an offering. Embracing what God does for you is the best thing you can do for him. Don't become so well-adjusted to your culture that you fit into it without even thinking. Instead, fix your attention on God. You'll be changed from the inside out. Readily recognize what he wants from you, and quickly respond to it. Unlike the culture around you, always dragging you down to its level of immaturity, God brings the best out of you, develops well-formed maturity in you.*

## Romans 12:2 (AMP)

*And do not be conformed to this world [any longer with its superficial values and customs], but be transformed and progressively changed [as you mature spiritually] by the renewing of your mind [focusing on godly values and ethical attitudes], so that you may prove [for yourselves] what the will of God is, that which is good and acceptable and perfect [in His plan and purpose for you].*

**Prayer Confession:** Lord, I recognize that the custom of this society leans toward being overindulgent, especially with food. However, I reject conforming to the culture around me which promotes unhealthy eating and offers foolish, ill-advised plans for weight loss. Instead I choose to fix my attention on You, and I choose to lean toward Your way of thinking and doing things, even when I'm frustrated or uncertain. Holy Spirit, You're directing and guiding me, so I don't have to worry about what happens next. I thank You, Father God, as I place my health and wellness efforts before you today, I am being transformed from the inside out! Your Word says You crown my efforts with success, so I boldly declare, "I am a success story!" In Jesus' name, Amen.

# DAY TWO
## SEE YOURSELF AS
## AN ATHLETE

When I was growing up, I spent almost
all of my summer breaks with my
grandparents in Alabama. I, particularly,
spent a lot of time with Grandmama,
who was my first best friend and was
basically a mix between Madea and
the Oracle from "The Matrix." Grandmama had a garden that I got to work
in with her. I was responsible for
pulling up cucumbers, squash, toma-

toes, turnips, and greens—like mustards and collards and something she called, "poke salad."

Besides the garden, Grandmama and Granddaddy also had a farm with cows, a bull, pigs, and guineas (fowl). Grandmama was super feisty, but she was very gentle with the animals. The cows would even eat out of her hands. Granddaddy had a building on the property where he would cure meats. On our way back to the house from the fields, Grandmama and I would gather eggs in one pouch pocket and black-berries in another.

My grandparents were rich. That is what I realize now. They were rich in that they were self-sufficient. They grew and raised their own food, so it was vital, they tended to the gardens and their farm.

I remember other folks in the community also grew some of their food but mostly herbs and tomatoes on the side of their houses. Looking back, I see those projects didn't seem to get the same attention that my grandparents gave to their gardens and their farm. If the neighbor's herbs and tomatoes did well, that was fine. If they didn't do well, that was fine, too. Tending to those plants was NOT a part of their everyday livelihood. Here's where I'm going with this: There is a difference in the mentality between a committed farmer or gardener versus the thinking of someone who is only experimenting with growing "stuff" on the side of the house.

When I consider what it means to be an athlete, I think about the fact an athlete is not someone who is just experimenting with eating healthier and works out when they feel up to it. Being an athlete is a different distinction. Athletes train. They don't try. The way they eat, workout, sleep, and think are almost always goal-oriented. Like Grandmama and Granddaddy, everything that happened in that garden and on that farm was part of a larger goal for the family. It was more than a hobby or a passing interest.

As we go forward on our weight-loss journeys, I think it matters that we begin to see ourselves like athletes.

This does not mean we have to work out for hours on end or count macros (macronutrients: carbohydrates, protein, and fat) for every meal. What it does mean; however, is we consider the thoughts, habits, and discipline of athletes and visualize ourselves as being just as capable of such a level of dedication. I rehearse and recite 1 Corinthians 9:27 as a habit. When I am done, I add to it saying, "I am an athlete!" It empowers my thinking and overpowers toxic thoughts that try to prevent me from achieving my goals.

Today, dabble in some research on articles and interviews about how athletes think. What are their habits? That, coupled with reading and meditating on 1 Corinthians 9:27, will lead you to the next step of your particular weight-loss journey—obtaining wisdom.

## I Corinthians 9:27 (NLT)

*I discipline my body like an athlete, training it to do what it should. Otherwise, I fear that after preaching to others I myself might be disqualified.*

## 1 Corinthians 9:27 (MSG)

*I don't know about you, but I'm running hard for the finish line. I'm giving it everything I've got. No sloppy living for me! I'm staying alert and in top condition. I'm not going to get caught napping, telling everyone else all about it and then missing out myself.*

**Prayer Confession:** Father God, in the name of Jesus, by Your Spirit, help me today to discipline my body like an athlete. Infuse me with the strength and might to train and eat in the way I should, so I may *prosper and be in health.* I need to fulfill the purpose and desires You've put in my heart. So, I don't want to vex my soul because of my own lack of self-control and end up in another spiral of self-sabotage. My hope is in You, Lord. Not in myself alone nor in any other person, plan, or program. Today, I boldly decree I am in optimum health! I'm in the best shape of my life right now, like an athlete! In Jesus' name, Amen.

# DAY THREE
## WISDOM FOR YOUR PARTICULAR WEIGHT-LOSS JOURNEY

Listen, there are so many plans and strategies and even tricks claiming to be the solution for weight woes. Sometimes, it can be confusing to know which fitness program (yoga, running, weight-training, group fitness, etc.) or eating style (paleo, keto, vegan, etc.) is the right one for our lifestyle and personality. God knows us better than we know ourselves. And, He knows what is the best pathway for YOU on this leg of your weight-loss journey. Just because you know someone who was successful with *Whole30* for example, or you saw something online about how some protein shake, skinny tea, pills, or potion worked for what seemed to be a miracle for someone else, that doesn't mean that's what the Lord would have you do. It can be tempting to just order *that* product, pay *that* Instagram coach, or join *that* challenge, so that you can get the results they are marketing. Perhaps, that is exactly what you should do but also be open to the idea that it may not be for you at all. Either way, be guided by wisdom and not by frustration.

In my own experience, the Holy Spirit inspired me to get educated about clean eating, meal prep, and weight training. I did not follow any of the weight-loss programs that we've come to know about. I don't have anything against programs, especially nutritionally sound ones. They just don't happen to be a part of MY testimony. Trust me, I definitely wondered about this because I tried programs in the past. But this time, I didn't want to rely on my own ideas, and I didn't want to consider what did or did not work in the past. I also didn't want to waste any money or time doing what seemed right. I needed to hear from God because I figured if He was leading, I would not be disappointed with the result.

For Day Three the focus is to ask God about what YOU need to do next. What meal plan should you use? Should you get a gym membership, hire a personal trainer, or work out at home? Should you join a sports league or a running club? Should you start out by ordering meal kits, or should you master creating healthy versions of your favorite dishes? Should you schedule a consultation for *that* procedure, or consider not having it at all? There are sooooo many ways to go about this. But, you just need THE particular way that is right for you because that's the way that will result in lasting transformation. It's the way that has God's grace available for you to see it through.

Let's ask for His wisdom. Even if you have already been on a particular plan, be open to new insight.

---

## James 1:5 (MSG)

*If you don't know what you're doing, pray to the Father. He loves to help. You'll get his help and won't be condescended to when you ask for it. Ask boldly, believingly, without a second thought. People who "worry their prayers" are like wind-whipped waves. Don't think you're going to get anything from the Master that way, adrift at sea, keeping all your options open.*

## James 1:5 (AMP)

*If any of you lacks wisdom [to guide him through a decision or circumstance], he is to ask of [our benevolent] God, who gives to everyone generously and without rebuke or blame, and it will be given to him.*

**Prayer Confession:** Father God, by Your Spirit, You are leading me into wisdom as it relates to decisions about the best ways for me to eat and work out. There are so many different plans and programs. Some I can recognize as crazy, but others seem sound. I desire to select the plan that will be ideal for me. Help me to discern which to choose. Open my eyes and ears to recognize Your answers as I go throughout the day. You are generous with Your wisdom. Keep me mindful that wisdom for weight-loss is available to me whenever I ask. I declare even now that I have it! I have weight-loss wisdom! In Jesus' name, Amen.

# DAY FOUR
## THE GRACE FACTOR

Y'all, sometimes I just don't get it. Like, for real. I have had days when my mind was racing with thoughts like:

- Why does this have to be my issue?
- Why couldn't I have been like those girls who can eat trash, don't work out, and still look photoshopped in real life?!
- Why can't I just do this once and for all, and it sticks?

- Why do I have to be so super intentional with my eating every single day?
- When is this gon' be over?!!! Jesus, can I borrow my "glorified body" for on earth?!

Topic change for a sec. I absolutely don't understand SnapChat. It's so bonkers to me. As a woman in my mid-40s, I see SnapChat as just a circus mirror that takes pictures. I just don't get it. I enjoy taking pictures of myself (which I never share) just to see what I'd look like as an electric bunny or whatever those things are. But, still, I just don't get it. I say that to say this. I don't get my "weight" thing either! Intellectually, I get it. I understand that consistency with clean eating, exercise, and proper rest leads to weight loss. But, I have complained to God and to myself in the mirror, that I don't get how it seems to be my "cross to bear." It has made me so frustrated and super annoyed at times! But, yet and still, it is the very thing the Holy Spirit has used over the past few years to teach and train me, have me uplift others, and in turn, uplift myself.

It's like He comforts and strengthens me when I reach out and share what I'm going through on my own journey. I've disqualified myself before, thinking I was in no position to help others when I myself am still a work in progress. The good news for us, as believers, is we are not limited by our own strength. Instead, we can be reassured by God's promise of strengthening us, energizing us, and even reigniting our desire and ability to fulfill our purpose (which absolutely includes being in good health) for HIS good pleasure. It's for His good pleasure. So, He would love to have you partner with Him on your weight-loss journey! We just need to ask. Let's do that now.

Philippians 2:13 (AMP)

*For it is [not your strength, but it is] God who is effectively at work in you, both to will and to work [that is, strengthening, energizing, and creating in you the longing and the ability to fulfill your purpose] for His good pleasure.*

**Prayer Confession:** Lord, thank You for Your grace. I am so grateful for how Your grace and Your mercy are always available to me in any situation and at any time. I need Your grace and mercy along this weight-loss journey. I recognize that even my best efforts don't seem like enough when I am operating simply off of willpower or some other source of motivation. So, I am asking You to be my supernatural coach! I will take courage in knowing You are effectively at work in me. You give me ideas and insight daily. You charge up my will, and You infuse me with the strength and energy I need to endure with enthusiasm. I receive it by faith. In Jesus' name, Amen.

# DAY FIVE
## THE RUDDER

Last summer, I did a talk with my *Wisdom for Weight-Loss* tribe about "the rudder." It's one of the many times where I am sharing a message to other people, but I'm really talking to myself. Whosoever can benefit from it, but I'm sho nuff talking to myself! Now, let me tell you what a "rudder" is. So, a rudder is the device that directs, governs, steers, or guides a ship/boat or aircraft. The rudder in our lives (what directs, governs, steers, or guides our choices) is basically our words—those words that fall out of our mouths as a result of our predominant thoughts.

This is important because during our weight-loss journey, we need to not only be purposeful about what we choose to put *in* our mouths but also about what we allow to come *out* of our mouths. We speak contrary to what we hope to accomplish when we say things like:

- "It doesn't seem like I'm making any real progress. I don't know if it matters anymore."
- "I always gain the weight back."
- "I don't know if I'll be able to keep this up and be consistent anyway."
- "I'm just not motivated."

I've said all of these things and far worse. I'm sharing this with you in case you can relate. Know that you're not the only one, and you can overcome that kind of toxic speaking and thinking. Speaking like this is dangerous and can produce just what you say. Which is more of what you don't want, right?

So, for Day Five, my prayer for us is that we abort that line of *tom-foolery* and instead be intentional about using our words to proclaim our success on this weight-loss journey. Whether it's looking like what we want or not. Because our rudder (the words we speak) can turn this thang around, y'all!

## Proverbs 18:21 (AMP)

*Death and life are in the power of the tongue, And those who love it and indulge it will eat its fruit and bear the consequences of their words.*

## James 3:4-6 (MSG)

*A bit in the mouth of a horse controls the whole horse. A small rudder on a huge ship in the hands of a skilled captain sets a course in the face of the strongest winds. A word out of your mouth may seem of no account, but it can accomplish nearly anything— or destroy it! It only takes a spark, remember, to set off a forest fire. A careless or wrongly placed word out of your mouth can do that.*

**Prayer Confession:** Father, God, in the name of Jesus, if I should say anything that actually opposes my victory, I thank You that You will correct me by Your Spirit! I desire to speak life concerning my health, so I may enjoy the fruit of confessing Your Word, versus speaking contrary to my faith and having to bear the consequences of those words. Thank You, Father, God for being concerned about every single thing that concerns me. My weight-loss journey is included in that, and I am so grateful.

# DAY SIX
## WILL POWER VS. HIS POWER

There is not a day that goes by that I don't have to be intentional concerning my health and wellness. Some days I'm like, "Yay, me!" And other days, I have to "Baby, -what-is-you-doing?" myself (as Issa Rae says) lol! Yet, even when I feel like I'm falling off, I'm still winning because...God.

I heard Dr. Bill Winston once say, "Deliverance is instant, but freedom is progressive." I never forgot that. It was years ago that I heard that. It still sticks with me. It reminds me, although the Lord has delivered me from the bondage of obesity and all the harassing spirits that accompany it, getting free and staying free is a whole different process. And, for me, as I said before, it's an everyday thing. Like, I'm so for real.

So, the scripture we're looking at for Day Six brings me such relief, y'all! It's good news to me because what I get from it is, I don't have to rely on my own strength. My own "will power" can be flaky and frail and funny acting. But according to the Word, God is working in us to strengthen and energize us, and He creates in us the longing and the ability to fulfill our purpose. His purpose for us includes us prospering in the area of our health! Because how are we going to be really effective, impactful, and available if our bodies are raggedy and tired all the time? Just saying.

## Philippians 2:13 (AMP)

*For it is [not your strength, but it is] God who is effectively at work in you, both to will and to work [that is, strengthening, energizing, and creating in you the longing and the ability to fulfill your purpose] for His good pleasure.*

## Philippians 2:13 (NLT)

*For God is working in you, giving you the desire and the power to do what pleases him.*

69

**Prayer Confession:** Lord, thank You for Your exceeding great and precious promises! By faith I take hold of Your Word that says You are working in me right now. YOU ARE STRENGTHENING ME, ENERGIZING ME, AND CREATING IN ME THE LONGING *AND* THE ABILITY TO FULFILL MY PURPOSE! I know my purpose includes prosperity in the area of health and wellness. And, I know faith pleases You. So, I put my faith in Your power and not in my own will power, as I walk out the freedom of a fit lifestyle. In Jesus' name, Amen.

# DAY SEVEN
## THE PURPOSE PART

Last summer, I took a class called "Deeper Discipleship," where I was learning more about how to practically apply the Word of God and about how to affirm who I am in Christ. During one of our Thursday night sessions, our teacher Dr. Jill, said, "It is a sad thing to have more purpose than health." I still am struck by that statement. I see it as a call to action to be purposeful on a daily basis regarding success in the area of physical health. Like, whoa. I get it in a new way now. THIS is why I must continue to encourage and share about the crucial connection between faith and fitness/ wellness/weight-loss, etc. It's very much a part of our purpose package!

Consider what you've been called to do. Your purpose. Your ultimate assignment. That dream that you are hoping to accomplish. That movement that is to come from you. The cultures and nations and industries and systems that will be transformed because of you. Now, imagine you being in optimum health to fulfill the tasks and having the vibrancy and stamina to meet the demands that your work and purpose call for. And, by the way, every time I say the word "you," I'm most certainly talking to myself first. We're in this thing together, y'all. So, for Day Seven let's pray for our success in prospering in our health. Our purpose (and that of others) depends on it!

### 3 John 2 (AMP)

*Beloved, I pray that in every way you may succeed and prosper and be in good health [physically], just as [I know] your soul prospers [spiritually].*

### 3 John 2 (NLT)

*Dear friend, I hope all is well with you and that you are as healthy in body as you are strong in spirit.*

**Prayer Confession:** In the name of Jesus, I confess that I am a success story already! I am prospering (flourishing and progressing) in my physical health. And, I am thriving in my mental health. I'm expanding in my mind, will, intellect, and emotions. Just as Your Word says, Father, I am as healthy in body as I am strong in spirit. I am in good health, and I am prospering spiritually.

# DAY EIGHT
## INTEGRITY IS THE MEASUREMENT NOT THE SCALE!

In 2011, I tried *Weight Watchers* (WW). My goal was just to reach two-hundred pounds. For me, that would be bliss! But at two hundred and one pounds, when I was closer than ever before, the weight-loss halted. I reached a plateau, and it seemed like nothing not even cutting my "points" in half, or severely reducing my calorie requirements, which I foolishly tried, would work. I was outdone.

So, every time I got on the scale, I wanted to cry. Actually, I wanted to throw that dang scale against the wall. And, y'all sometimes I just cried after seeing that number. Then, I'd go look at myself in the mirror, so I could see just how pitiful I looked. No pity party is complete without looking at yourself crying in the mirror, right? Well, after weeks of this battle with the scale, I started to feel like it didn't matter anymore. Maybe I was just meant to be a big girl. And, it was okay, because I was cute and smart and funny. So, I should just deal with it. But, deep down, that's not what I really wanted.

Looking back, I realize *Weight Watchers* was not the problem. Because, although I'm not a member of WW now, but I know it works if you work it. Any plan, whether wise or cray-cray, works if you are consistent with it. That's just science. The REAL problem was I did not trust I could be successful. My fears of failing again overwhelmed me. So, when I didn't see progress in the way I had hoped, it was easy to give up. Again. I had trained my spirit to quit. And, as a consequence, I would pick up every single pound that I dropped and put it right back on. It was a vicious cycle.

I lacked integrity in my weight-loss journey. I'm using the word *integrity* here to mean—keeping your word. Doing what is right just because it's right no matter who is watching. And, for me it also means being constant. Regardless of distractions and adversities.

Fast forward to the summer of 2014. I started going through a major transformation from the inside out. As it pertained to my wellness, I began to make small goals for myself each week. For example, I would set a fitness goal to go for a walk for thirty minutes, four days out of the week. And, I'd make a nutrition goal, such as making one of my daily meals, a salad, with a new vegetable. At the end of each week, I measured my success NOT by what that dang scale reported, but I was now measuring my success by whether or not I accomplished the things I said I would do. If I kept my word to myself, then it was a victory. Integrity was the scale.

These integrity victories began to replace my dependency on the scale, which interestingly started to slowly move in my favor. But, even when the scale seemed unfriendly, I had the inspiration to keep going because of all the other victories I was amassing through keeping my word to myself.

This is why for Day Eight I want us to pray that our integrity will be developed, and that this integrity will keep us on track during the different phases of our weight-loss journey.

P.S. It's noble to keep your word to others during your weight-loss journey —your trainer, your workout buddies, your accountability partner. But, it's just as honorable to keep your word to yourself.

You know how we do. Read the scriptures. Pray the scriptures.

Proverbs 11:3 (NIV)

*The integrity of the upright guides them, but the unfaithful are destroyed by their duplicity.*

Proverbs 11:3a (MSG)

*The integrity of the honest keeps them on track.*

**Prayer Confession:** Father, God, in the name of Jesus, I know You desire that I prosper in my health. I acknowledge in order to do that, I need Your grace and strength to be able to demonstrate integrity in my weight-loss journey. Your Word says *integrity can be a guide for me and keep me on track.* I need Your help to keep my word to myself, Lord. By faith, I profess I am a person of integrity, especially in my relationship to myself. I do what I say I will do. I eat clean this week just like I've said I would. I exercise this week just like I've said I would. And, I hydrate myself and get proper rest just like I've been saying I would. In Jesus' name, Amen!

# DAY NINE
## IT'S THE CLIMB

I used to work for *Disney Cruise Lines*. Y'all, I cannot count how many times I had to endure the "Hannah Montana the Movie" soundtrack while working with the Youth Entertainment Team. However, one song, in particular, always moved me. It was the song, "The Climb."

I thought of "The Climb" just now as I was staring at one of the goal boards I keep in the corner of my living room. I made that board in January, 2014. I had just gotten down to two hundred and thirty-seven pounds, down from two hundred and forty-six, the previous year. So, with fresh motivation, I set a goal weight of one hundred and forty-two—my college freshman weight. At the time I set that goal, it was audacious to say the least. But, as much as I felt so far from it, I dared to put it up anyway. I was in a mindset where I was finally determined no matter how long it took, I was going to get there. No more time lines based on superficial things like birthdays, events, or vacations. That used to be a big thingfor me. The way I called myself planning it is laughable now. I can tell you how I got over that!

I got frustrated setting these deadlines and then never meeting them. I would beat myself up over it. Feel miserable. But, then, just repeat the same insane process. I know some would say it's good to set deadlines. I, however, even hate the sound of the word *dead*lines. So, I let that go. I just wanted to make some progress. Whenever that was, as long as it was progress, that was gon' be cool with me. I was still figuring out how to measure success (the scale would turn out to NOT be the answer as you discovered in Day Eight), but what I did figure out, is that the "climb" needed more appreciation than I had given it.

The "climb," in my view, is the daily experience of it all, and the mental/emotional/spiritual adventures that go along with it, too. Sometimes, it feels like smooth sailing, other times it feels more like a ride on the *Crazy Train* with stops to the *Emotional Roller Coaster*. All that matters though! All that is part of your testimony, honey. During the "climb," our faith is producing endurance. And, we need endurance, don't we?! And, that endurance is producing character, which is leading to ultimate freedom in this area of health for us.

So, yeah. As the song says, "Ain't about how fast I get there...It's the climb!" I'm still climbing, y'all, and I am trying to be mindful to appreciate the experience. For Day Nine let's pray for the faith to keep climbing toward our goals. Whether you want to run a marathon, fit back into your favorite dress or suit, wear a bikini this summer, or actually climb a whole mountain, let's give it up for the scenic route!

## Romans 5:3-5 (NLT)

*³ We can rejoice, too, when we run into problems and trials, for we know that they help us develop endurance.⁴ And endurance develops strength of character, and character strengthens our confident hope of salvation.⁵ And this hope will not lead to disappointment. For we know how dearly God loves us, because he has given us the Holy Spirit to fill our hearts with his love.*

**Prayer Confession:** Father God, in the name of Jesus, I am choosing to adjust my thinking about the challenges I face in my weight-loss journey. I agree with Your Word which says, I can *rejoice when I run into problems and trials because those things can help me develop endurance.* Your Word tells me *endurance develops strength of character* in me. Strength of character produces greater confidence and hope in You. And, when I have my hope in You (not in myself or in any program or plan or person), I will NOT end up in disappointment. Thank You for the victories my special climb is leading me to. In Jesus' name, Amen.

# DAY TEN
## THINK HIGHLY OF YOURSELF

I've been asked where my "aha" moment came from. Looking back, I can see that it was birthed out of a very broken place. I felt so hopeless in so many different areas of my life. Y'all, it was like everything was in "transition!" From my career, to my housing situation, to finances, to family, and to transportation...just everything seemed to be unraveling! I'm not at all saying your life has to be raggedy in order for real change to come. What I am saying is, the situation I found myself in, I felt like the only thing I could control was the things related to my identity.

While on a walk one summer morning in 2014, I decided I would be more compassionate with myself and treat myself as if I were my own best friend. I would be good to myself in every way. That included the way I talked to myself about myself. Now, trust. This was a slow, super slow, snail slow process! I had a history of negative self-talk, and my faith was sooooo contaminated by fear and insecurity to the degree that I would beat myself up over little common mishaps, such as losing my keys. Anyway, I set out to reset my thinking by replacing pitiful thoughts with powerful ones. Affirming myself. Not just saying affirmations, though. But, proclaiming what the Word of God says about me. There is power in the Word! Y'all already know.

Here's something else: The Lord wants us to think highly of ourselves! *He* thinks highly of us, so we should, too. Now, creating this as a habit was like mental gymnastics for me, y'all. Like, I would have to replace my negative thoughts continually! If I said something like, "I just can't seem to get this right," then I would be convicted in the depths of my soul to fix that immediately. It was as if the Holy Spirit was saying, "What did you say???" Then, I'd switch it up real fast. I prayed to have that level of conviction. I didn't want to be comfortable, content, or immune to speaking harshly to myself or about my future.

For Day Ten, let's commit to agreeing with God and affirming ourselves with the Word. There are sooooo many scriptures you can choose to start this process. I'll just share one for now. Keep building your list, though! It matters so much. Otherwise, weight loss can seem like a mental maze!

Psalm 139:14 (NLT)

*Thank you for making me so wonderfully complex! Your workmanship is marvelous—how well I know it.*

Psalm 139:14 (MSG)

*I thank you, High God—you're breathtaking! Body and soul, I am marvelously made! I worship in adoration—what a creation!*

**Prayer Confession:** Father, God, in the name of Jesus, help me to see myself through Your eyes, and let this new view include my being able to appreciate the way I look. The way I look even now! I don't need to wait to acknowledge my beauty. You've already made me marvelous inside and out! Your workmanship is wonderful! Lord, I praise You for how You made me. Help me to be able to think highly of myself like You already do. In Jesus' name, Amen.

# DAY ELEVEN
## SEEING YOURSELF AS A SUCCESS STORY NOW!

It was very helpful for me to write out my transformation story. From the start, that was my way of forecasting the change I wanted to see. And, I'm reminded of *Habakkuk 2* with practicing this because it is about the promise and power of having clarity around your vision. I STILL do this even now, actually! I write a narrative of what I have achieved before I achieve it. My lock screen and home screen on my phone have images that remind me of what I'm going to experience. Sometimes, I catch myself in a "Wait. Is this real?" moment because it seems so real in my mind even though the manifestation is still unfolding.

Like you, I've read plenty of success stories, so I have an idea of how a transformation story usually flows. I invite you to write out your own transformation story *before* it's fully experienced. Then, read it out loud. And, throughout your journey, take a look at it to remind yourself where you're headed. When I first did this exercise, I had no idea that my story would one day be shared by online magazines and print publications to inspire others in their weight-loss journeys. Perhaps, you will one day soon be sharing your story with the world, too!

Here's some prompts to help guide your thinking as you write your transformation story:

- What was your breakthrough moment —the moment you realized you had to make changes?
- Were you always overweight? If so, was it common in your family to have overweight family members?
- Were you ever athletic? If so, what sports or activities did you do?
- Have you stopped being athletic? If so, why do you think that is?
- What role do you think diet had in your weight gain?

- What kind of things did you used to eat?
- Was eating a way of coping for you? If so, what were you trying to soothe in your life?
- Once you realized you needed to make changes, what was the very first thing you did to begin your journey?
- Did you set any goals? What were they?
- Did you enlist help from a friend, family member, or fitness professional (like a personal trainer or nutritionist)?
- Did you join a gym? If so, what was your initial experience there?
- What sort of exercise did you do at first (i.e. strength training, cardio, Zumba etc.) and how was your experience with that?

- What changes did you make to your diet and nutrition program?
- What was the hardest part about changing your eating habits?
- Do you have any role models in life or on social media that helped you?
- What can you do now, physically that you could not do before?
- What is your next fitness or wellness goal?
- What do you do when you come face-to-face with some of your old food vices?
- What is one of your new favorite healthy recipes?
- Do you have any mantras or affirmations that you'd like to share?
- What advice would you give someone who has a lot of weight to lose?

## Habakkuk 2:2-3 (GWT)

*Then the Lord answered me, "Write the vision. Make it clear on tablets so that anyone can read it quickly. The vision will still happen at the appointed time. It hurries toward its goal. It won't be a lie. If it's delayed, wait for it. It will certainly happen. It won't be late."*

## Habakkuk 2:2-3 (NLT)

*"Write my answer plainly on tablets, so that a runner can carry the correct message to others. This vision is for a future time. It describes the end, and it will be fulfilled. If it seems slow in coming, wait patiently, for it will surely take place. It will not be delayed."*

## Prayer Confession:

Lord, by Your Spirit, You have given me a vision for how prospering in my health is connected to my purpose. Through wisdom, I have planned and written a strategy to help me achieve my goals. As I walk it out, I trust that You will be leading and guiding me along the best route to my "expected end" in this area of my life. When progress seems slow, help me not to give up or compare myself to others. Lord, I will be patient with myself. Thank You that you are always so patient with me. In Jesus' name, Amen.

# DAY TWELVE
## FEELING WEAK
## IS NOT WEAKNESS!!

As I mentioned before, in 2011, I joined *Weight Watchers*. It was my birthday present to myself to join the program. I was very excited and hopeful! By the way, this is not a plug for *Weight Watchers*. I'm not promoting it, and neither am I against it. But, I digress. One week, while in the program, I was more disciplined and diligent than I had ever been with my eating and working out. I couldn't wait to see my results at the weigh-in. Whelp, to my shock and disappointment, I had not lost a single pound. Instead, I had gained about two pounds!

This was long before I had any under-standing about the science of weight loss. And, long before I had gained some sanity about not being ruled by the number on the scale. So, at that time, seeing those results put me right on the crazy train, with a scheduled stop for the emotional roller coaster! I felt as if all my efforts had been in vain. And, I felt like it didn't matter anymore if I stuck with the program or not because losing weight must clearly be something that I could never do. An inventory of my thoughts went some-thing like this:

- Why am I successful in other areas but still struggling with my weight?

- Maybe I should just have weight-loss surgery. Oh wait...I can't afford that.

- Maybe I should just get comfortable with being a big girl.

- No one will probably care if I show up again at WW or at the gym anyway. Bet they won't even notice.

- I don't know if I can keep this up. I would probably just gain back any weight I lose anyway.

- Why do other people seem to lose weight so quickly and easily, but it's so hard for me and is taking forever?

- It doesn't matter how hard I try.

I know somebody can relate to at least one, if not all, of those thoughts. Maybe, you've entertained such thoughts as recently as today. It feels so real when you're in the thick of those thoughts. But, what I know now but didn't apply then is this, when we are at our weakest, THAT is when we are prime candidates for a strength infusion! When I was working out and eating healthy but relying on my own will power, I always ran out of steam at some point. Will-power is not strong enough to yank us out of a pit of pity. Motivational quotes and affirmations are nice and everything, but those exercises are limited by the mental or emotional state we're in when we say them. We can say an affirmation and be totally disconnected to believing it's true for us. We may as well be saying, "Twinkle, Twinkle, little star." The real transformation comes by drawing strength from GOD (through His Word and through prayer) whenever you start to feel weak on your journey. That is how you regain the ability and energy you need to keep going. His Word accomplishes what it is sent out to do. When you pray God's Word, it makes power available to you to do what you couldn't do before.

You are not failing on your weight-loss journey because you have those times when you feel weak. You are winning on your weight-loss journey because when you do feel weak, you now draw from God's strength. You are no longer limited to your own strength. You are strong in the Lord!

One more thing; we never plan to feel weak. It's one of those things that might just creep up on us. So, we have to be prepared in advance. Part of that preparation includes meditating (reading repeatedly, memorizing, saying aloud, singing, musing, pondering, etc.) a scripture like the one below. That Word will take root in your heart. Then, by the Spirit, you will be reminded of it and strengthened by it—just when you need it.

## 2 Corinthians 12:10b (AMP)

*When I am weak [in human strength], then I am strong [truly able, truly powerful, truly drawing from God's strength].*

## 2 Corinthians 12:10b (GWT)

*It's clear that when I'm weak, I am strong.*

**Prayer Confession:** I am grateful AND relieved I don't have to rely solely on my own strength, motivation, or smarts. My body and mind can get tired. And, there are times when I might go from being completely inspired to feeling like I'm on an emotional roller coaster. So, I thank You, Lord for Your promise that says, "When I am weak in human strength, then I am strong in You." I ask You, Holy Spirit, that when I am questioning if I'll be successful or not, You will bring to my remembrance that I am truly able and truly powerful when I am drawing from Your strength. I AM TRULY ABLE AND TRULY POWERFUL WHEN I AM DRAWING FROM YOUR STRENGTH! In Jesus' name, Amen.

One last thing...

The Lord is concerned about everything that concerns you. So, if you are concerned about your health, He certainly is. Because He wants the best for you anyway! As you are on this wellness journey now, know that our God is eager to have you ask Him to be your personal trainer, nutritionist, and your complete make-over specialist from the inside out! Invite Him in, sincerely, to do just that. You have discovered you need more than meal ideas, workout plans, and fitness challenges to lose the weight you desire to lose. At this point in your life, you know all about that stuff. And, what you don't know, you do know how to Google it. What we need is wisdom. What we need is to hear from

God on this. What we need is to be able to apply our faith to our daily efforts of doing the work to lose weight. What we shall have is *supernatural weight loss.* The *natural* part you will continue to pursue. That is the fitness and nutrition aspect of the process. The *super* part is where God steps in and empowers us to do what we could not do before in our own strength. The father of my faith, Dr. Bill Winston, likes to say, "God wants to put His super on your natural!"

Our willpower, motivation, and elaborate affirmations are nice, needful resources. But, those things do not have the power to maintain our deliverance from the unproductive, toxic, and dysfunctional thoughts and habits that have led us to an inflated weight in the first place.

Continue to read and meditate on the scripture passages. Look up other translations as well. Say the Word-based prayer confessions out loud. Hear yourself. Faith comes by hearing. I'll be doing them with you! Let's join our faith together and reach our wellness and weight-loss goals!

Love,
Q.

## *ABOUT THE AUTHOR*

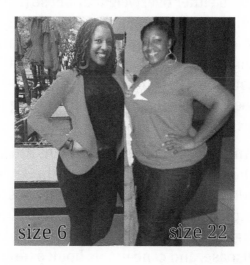

size 6        size 22

Queing Jones is a P.E. teacher, wellness blogger, nutrition curriculum writer, encouragement enthusiast, and author of the new devotional *Running in Church Can't Count for Cardio: 12 Practical Prayers to Ignite Your Weight-Loss Journey.*

Having had a lifetime experience with being either overweight or obese (from childhood through the age of forty), Queing has a uniquely empathetic and engaging voice that shines through in her newest collection of prayers on seeking the wisdom of God for weight-loss success.

Minister and psychologist, Dr. Anitra Shelton-Quinn says, "Given the grave public health threat that obesity poses, with links to chronic diseases including high blood pressure, cardiovascular disease, and cancer, this book extends a lifeline to those wanting to live a healthy, abundant life, for the Glory of God."

Queing enjoys riding her bike along Chicago's lake front, and she has no shame in being a savage in the game of Scrabble.

Join Queing's tribe of "Running Buddies!"

Blog: RunningInChurch.com

Instagram: @Wisdom4WeightLoss

Facebook: @Wisdom4WeightLoss

# About ZION Publishing House

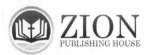

ZION Publishing House is a family-owned publishing company based in Washington, DC and South Dakota. ZION helps Christian authors tell their stories by providing an affordable alternative to traditional publishing. Our mission is to maintain a platform that educates and empowers independent Christian authors. We do this by cultivating talent in the inspirational and self-help genres for novice and experienced authors. The path to publishing can be daunting and extremely complex. We take pride in taking our clients by the hand and walking them through the publishing process to ensure they not only have a high-quality product that resonates with the reader, but they understand the many facets of the publishing industry and what it means to be a published author.

If you are a writer looking for an affordable path to high-quality publishing, visit our website at **www.zionpublishinghouse.com** to learn more.